Diving into Natural Dog Feeding:
A Fresh Start

S.Goldstein

Dedication

To all my fur-children, who have trotted through the corridors of my life, wagging their tails, and in their own unique ways, teaching me the real meaning of joy. Thank you, each one of you, for your unbounded love and the sunshine you've brought into my life. Thank you Muttley, Oliver, Bill, Brigitte and her litter, Alf, Afro, Coquito, Mimi, Rutherford, Hugo, Biquinhos de Lacre, Piu-Piu, Abby, Luna, Sky, Raven, and Tina. Your names are forever etched in my heart and your paw prints linger in my soul. In each wag, woof, and loving gaze, you have written the chapters of my happiness.

Acknowledgments

As I sit down to pen these acknowledgments, I am struck by the immense gratitude that fills my heart. This book, the experiences it contains, and the lessons it imparts wouldn't have been possible without the support and guidance of a remarkable group of people and, of course, one very special Westie, Muttley.

First and foremost, my utmost appreciation goes to my furry companion, who embarked on this natural food journey with me, teaching me valuable lessons. His patience, resilience, and ever-wagging tail have been the driving force behind this book.

A heartfelt thank you to Dr. Elisabeth, our trusted veterinarian, whose wealth of knowledge and dedication to canine health has been invaluable. Her guidance and willingness to answer my countless questions greatly influenced our transition to natural dog food.

I am immensely grateful to my family and friends who, despite their initial skepticism, embraced our new approach to canine nutrition. Their encouragement and participation in taste-testing new recipes brought much joy to this journey.

I must express my gratitude to the numerous authors, researchers, and bloggers in the field of canine nutrition whose work has been a vital source of knowledge and inspiration. Their diligence in uncovering and sharing information about natural dog food has paved the way for dog owners like myself.

I also greatly thank my editor, whose keen eye and insightful suggestions have shaped this book into a guide that I hope will significantly help other dog owners.

Lastly, I'd like to thank you, the readers, for picking up this book and showing an interest in the health and happiness of your canine companion. Our story can inspire you to explore the wonderful world of natural dog food and experience the joy and benefits it can bring to your furry friend. With the most profound appreciation, Simone and Muttley.

Contents

Introduction - The Beginning Of Our Journey

Before diving into our journey toward natural dog food, we must share a bit about who we are. My name is Simone, and the star of our tale is my beloved West Highland Terrier, affectionately known as Muttley. A ball of Muttley has been my constant companion and source of joy for several years; a ball of energy with a white, furry coat and a heart full of love begins much like any other pet owner's. Our usual routine was morning walks, playtimes, cuddles, and the traditional commercial dog food diet. Kibble and canned food were staples in Muttle's diet, mainly because of their convenience and the widespread belief that they provided complete dog nutrition.

I remember the day Muttley looked up at me with those gleaming eyes, crunching on his kibble without the slightest idea that his dietwould change dramatically. As a loving pet parent, my primary concern has always been his well-being. Little did I know then that my quest to ensure his excellent health would lead us down a less-traveled path filled with wholesome foods and a completely fresh approach to his nutrition.

My introduction to natural dog food was purely coincidental. One day, I stumbled upon an article that discussed the benefits of natural,homemade food for dogs. Intrigued, I started researching, reading more articles, watching documentaries, and even reaching out to veterinarians and other dog owners who had ventured down this path.

The more I discovered about natural dog food, the more I became convinced that this was a journey worth taking. There was a whole world beyond the shelves of processed pet food, and I felt drawn toexplore it for Muttley's health and happiness.

However, the path to natural dog food was not strewn with roses. It involved making tough decisions, investing more time and energy, overcoming hurdles, and, most importantly, staying committed to the cause even when things got tough. But every step and challenge was worth the improvement I saw in his health and vitality.

This book is an account of our journey. A testament to our shared experiences, the ups and downs, the trials, and triumphs, and ultimately, the wonderful world of natural dog food that we've cometo embrace.

Whether you're a seasoned pet parent or a new dog owner, I hope our story provides insights, answers some questions, and inspires youto explore natural dog food for your furry friend. After all, every journey begins with a single step, and this was ours. Let's embark on this adventure together.

1 Unearthing The Truth About Commercial Dog Food

The story of our journey towards natural dog food begins with the commonly used, commercially produced dog food we've all come to recognize. These are the bags of kibble and cans of wet food that line the shelves of pet stores and supermarkets. As a devoted pet owner, I had always assumed these foods were nutritionally complete and ideal for my dog. After all, they were marketed as 'complete and balanced,' containing everything my dog needed to thrive. However, after delving deeper into the subject, I discovered more of the story.

Unearthing the truth about commercial dog food was both complex and challenging. It began with me noticing subtle changes in my dog's health and energy levels. Despite being on a diet of top-rated commercial food, he seemed lethargic, his coat was dull, and he didn't seem his usual self. This observation led me to start questioning the quality and nutritional value of his food.

With extensive research, I learned that commercial dog food, while convenient, often needs to provide optimal nutrition for our furry friends. Many commercial foods are laden with fillers like corn, wheat, and soy, which offer little nutritional value. They are also often high in carbohydrates, an ingredient that dogs, as primarily carnivorous creatures, don't need in large quantities.

Moreover, the processing methods used in commercial pet food production can diminish ingredients' nutritional value. Essential nutrients can be lost during cooking and drying processes, with synthetic vitamins and minerals added back in later to compensate.

Additionally, many commercial dog foods contain additives and preservatives to increase shelf-life. Some of these substances have been linked to adverse health effects in dogs, ranging from allergiesand inflammation to more severe health conditions.

Upon uncovering these truths, I was shocked and felt a sense of guilt for not having known better. However, I also knew this was a turningpoint. I resolved to make a change and ensure my dog was getting themost nutritious diet possible, a decision that ultimately led us down the path toward natural dog food.

Unearthing the truth about commercial dog food was a pivotal moment in our journey, highlighting the importance of vigilance in what we feed our pets. It began a much-needed change and opened the door to a new, healthier lifestyle for my dog.

In the next chapter, we'll delve into the concept of natural dog food,what it entails, and why I consider it a viable alternative for my dog'sdietary needs.

2 Understanding Natural Dog Food: A Shift In Perspective

Before we delve deeper into my journey and the advantages of naturaldog food, it's essential to understand what natural dog food truly means and why it signifies a critical shift in perspective for any pet owner.

'Natural dog food' refers to meals prepared using fresh, whole, and minimally processed ingredients. Natural dog food primarily consists of proteins (like meat or fish), vegetables, fruits, and sometimes whole grains. The ingredients used are as close to their natural state as possible, without artificial preservatives, colors, or flavors.

Understanding natural dog food requires us to reevaluate how we perceive pet nutrition. Many dog owners, including myself initially, might be under the impression that commercial dog foods are the best nutrition source for our canine companions. After all, these foods are prepared by experts, right? This perspective, though commonplace, is gradually being challenged as we discover more about canine nutrition.

By exploring natural dog food, we understand that our dogs' nutritional requirements aren't so different from our own. Dogs, like humans, benefit from a varied diet that includes high-quality proteins, a range of vegetables and fruits, and balanced fats. Natural dog food provides this in a form closer to what dogs might have eaten in the wild.

However, the shift in perspective comes with its challenges. The commercial pet food industry is well-established; moving away from it can take time and effort. Yet, as we'll discover in the upcoming chapters, the rewards outweigh these challenges significantly.

Transitioning to natural dog food involves more than changing what goes into our dogs' bowls. It's a shift in understanding that our dogs deserve food that is as minimally processed, wholesome, and nutritionally rich as we'd like to feed ourselves. It's about recognizing that our furry friends, who give us so much unconditional love, deserve the best possible nourishment we can provide.

As we progress in this book, you'll learn more about my experience navigating this shift, my challenges, and how it ultimately made a significant difference in my dog's life and health.

But before we dive into the nitty-gritty of this transition, let's first explore why commercial dog food might not be the best choice for our pets, a realization that initially sparked my journey toward natural dog food. The next chapter will shed light on this topic, laying the groundwork for understanding why this shift in perspective is beneficial and necessary.

3 The Big Transition: My Dog's First Steps Towards Natural Food

It was not one fine morning when I decided to shift my dog to a natural diet. It was a gradual decision influenced by countless hours of research, consultations with veterinarians, and a growing concern aboutthe long-term health impacts of commercial dog food. It was time for abig transition.

But change, as we know, is never easy - and this was no exception.

In the beginning, there was skepticism, not just from my family members, who were worried about the feasibility and practicality of theidea, but also from my dear canine companion. After years of being fed commercial dog food, he needed to be more confident about this new culinary experience. His first few encounters with natural food were met with curious sniffs, cautious licks, and many unsure glances my way.

The first few days were filled with trial and error. Some recipes were met with enthusiasm, others with downright disapproval. I quickly learned that while my Westie loved sweet potatoes and chicken, he didnot like quinoa or kale. It was like deciphering a new language of love, health, and well-being that I was eager to master.

I also realized that while natural dog food provided many health benefits, a balanced diet was crucial. It was more complex than feedingmy dog a medley of fresh meats, fruits, and vegetables. I needed to ensure he was getting the right proportions of protein, carbohydrates, fats, vitamins, and minerals. Consulting with a pet nutrition expert was incredibly helpful during this phase, and I highly recommend this to anyone considering the shift.

Gradually, as weeks turned into months, my Westie and I started getting comfortable with this new routine. His initial skepticism turnedinto anticipation and joy every mealtime. I could see the excitement in his eyes, his wagging tail every time I prepared his food.

Looking back, the transition to natural dog food was not a walk in the park, but witnessing the positive changes it brought about in my Westie made it worth every hurdle. It was more than just about feeding him differently; it was about embracing a new lifestyle prioritizing health, wellness, and a deeper understanding of my dog's needs.

The big transition was a journey of transformation, bonding, andlearning that brought us closer.

4 Overcoming Hurdles: Challenges Of The Shift To Natural Diet

Transitioning to a natural diet for your dog may sound straightforward, but like any significant change, it comes with its own challenge. While I watched my dog reaps the benefits of this wholesome diet over time; getting there was not a walk in the park. This chapter is about our obstacles and how we overcame them, hoping our experience can makeyour journey smoother.

4.1 Uncertainty and Skepticism

When I first started considering a natural diet for my furry friend, I wasmet with a wave of skepticism from various quarters - friends, family, and even some vets. Many people warned me about the possible nutritional deficiencies or the risks of feeding my dog the wrong types of food. But instead of letting these concerns discourage me, I turned them into a motivating factor to learn more and ensure I was doing theright thing for my dog.

4.2   Dealing with Information Overload

In this age of the internet, there's no shortage of information, and when I began my research on natural dog food, I was overwhelmed. Reading articles, studies, and forums took time to find reliable, science-backed information. I found it helpful to stick to reputable sources and consult with a holistic vet or a pet nutritionist to navigate the sea of information.

4.3 Meal Preparation and Time Management

Meal preparation for a dog on a natural diet takes more time and effortthan simply pouring kibble into a bowl. Initially, it felt like a daunting task. However, with some planning and shortcuts - like meal prepping in bulk and freezing individual portions - it became manageable, even with my busy schedule.

4.4 **Managing the Cost**

Natural dog food can be more expensive than commercial dog food, depending on the ingredients used. I needed to balance choosing high- quality, nutritious ingredients and staying within my budget. Shopping seasonally, buying in bulk, and using a mix of premium and budget- friendly but still nutritious ingredients helped manage the cost.

4.4   Monitoring Health and Adjustments

Every dog is unique, and what works for one might not work for another. After transitioning to natural food, I had to closely monitor my dog's health - checking his weight, energy levels, and coat condition regularly. Initially, we had to adjust the proportions of different ingredients several times to meet her specific needs.

Switching to a natural diet for my dog was a journey with a few stumbling blocks. However, seeing the positive changes in her health and vitality made every challenge worthwhile. This chapter aims to help you anticipate and prepare for potential difficulties, making your transition as smooth as possible.

Transitioning to a natural diet isn't always easy, but it is an enriching journey. I hope our experiences can shed some light on the path for you.

5 Tips And Tricks: Preparing Natural Dog Food At Home

As we journey toward natural dog food, a common question arises: How can we best prepare meals at home? This chapter offers practical advice and effective techniques to help you confidently transition to homemade, natural dog food.

First, it's vital to understand that our furry friends need a balanced diet like us. A diet consisting exclusively of chicken and rice, for example, lacks the variety of nutrients dogs need. Ideally, your dog's diet should include a mixture of fruits, vegetables, and complex carbohydrates. A good rule of thumb is that protein should make up about 40% of your dog's meal, with the remaining 60% being a mix of fruits, vegetables, and grains.

One essential tip is to prepare your dog's meals in large batches to save time. Cook the food thoroughly, let it cool, and then portion it into daily servings. You can store these servings in the fridge if you plan to use them in the next few days or freeze them for more extended storage. Remember, variety ensures your pet gets all the necessary nutrients.

Gradually avoid upsetting their stomach when introducing new foods to your dog's diet. Start by replacing a small portion of their usual fare with fresh ingredients and the quantity over a week or so.

Keep an eye out for changes in your dog's behavior or physical condition after introducing new foods. Dogs, like people, can have food allergies or sensitivities. Symptoms include scratching, paw licking, ear infections, or gastrointestinal issues. You should consult your vet immediately if you notice any of these signs.

Always ensure that the food you feed your dog is safe for canine consumption. Some perfectly safe foods for humans can be toxic to dogs, including chocolate, grapes, raisins, onions, garlic, and xylitol (a common sweetener).

Make mealtime fun and enriching by using food puzzles or slow feeders. This can help engage your dog's mind and slow their eating, particularly for dogs that gulp their food.

Remember, transitioning to homemade, natural dog food is a journey, not a destination. It will take time and patience. Be encouraged if your dog is initially hesitant or if you encounter challenges along the way. With time, patience, and persistence, you can provide your best friend with nourishing meals that contribute to their overall health and well-being.

As you progress on this journey, remember that your veterinarian is an invaluable resource. Always consult with them before making significant changes to your dog's diet.

In the next chapter, we will discuss some of my dog's favorite homemade, natural recipes, which have been a hit in our home. This will give you a starting point for your homemade dog food journey.

Stay tuned, and remember - every small step you take is a giant leap toward ensuring the health and happiness of your beloved pet.

6 Tail-Wagging Recipes: My Dog's Favorite Natural Dishes

In this chapter, we will delve into the culinary delights that have not only delighted my dog but also supported his health and wellness.

These recipes have been developed and adapted based on my dog's taste preferences and nutritional needs. So, let's dive in and whip up some scrumptious meals for our furry friends!

Recipe 1: Chicken and Vegetable Medley

One of my dog's all-time favorites, this dish is packed with protein and a colorful array of vegetables. It includes chicken breast, carrots, peas, sweet potatoes, and a sprinkle of olive oil for that extra dose of healthy fats. The beauty of this dish lies in its simplicity. It's easy to prepare, and my dog loves it!

Recipe 2: Fish Fiesta

This recipe is an excellent source of Omega-3 fatty acids essential for a healthy coat and skin. This dish is both nutritious and delicious and made with fresh salmon, cooked quinoa, and a mix of zucchini and bell peppers. I serve it slightly warmly, and my dog gobbles it every time!

Recipe 3: Beefy Brown Rice

If your dog is a fan of red meat, then this dish will be a hit. This recipe features lean ground beef, brown rice, and mixed vegetables like peas and carrots. The lean meat provides ample protein, while the brown rice offers wholesome fiber. It's hearty, balanced, and a favorite during the colder months.

Recipe 4: Turkey and Pumpkin Stew

This dish combines lean ground turkey and pumpkin puree for a festive and highly digestible meal, perfect for the fall season. I like adding some cooked quinoa for an extra punch of protein and fiber. It's a comforting stew that's loved by dogs and owners alike!

When preparing these dishes, please remember to keep seasoning to a minimum. Dogs don't require added salt or spices in their food, and certain seasonings can even be harmful. Always check with your vet if you need clarification about introducing a new food into your dog's diet.

Also, remember that every dog is different, and dietary needs vary based on age, breed, size, and health conditions. These recipes are meant to be a starting point and can be adjusted to meet the specific needs of your furry friend.

As you can see, preparing natural meals for your dog can be a fun and rewarding experience. It's all about knowing your dog's dietary needs, using fresh, wholesome ingredients, and adding a dash of love!

Remember, balance and variety are the keys to a successful transition to natural food. Try different recipes, rotate proteins and veggies, and observe your dog's reactions. The wag of a tail at mealtime will be a sure sign that you're on the right track.

In the next chapter, we'll discuss the health benefits I noticed in my dog after transitioning to natural dog food. Stay tuned!

7 Notable Improvements: Health Benefits Of Natural Dog Food

When I first embarked on the journey to switch my beloved canine companion to a natural diet, I did so with excitement and trepidation. I had read about the potential benefits, but would I see them firsthand? As it turns out, the answer was a resounding yes. The changes in my dog's health, energy, and overall well-being were terrific.

Improved Coat Condition

One of the most immediately noticeable changes was my dog's coat quality. His fur became glossier, softer, and healthier. While he had previously suffered from occasional bouts of dry, flaky skin, these instances significantly decreased with the introduction of natural foods. I attribute this to many raw food ingredients' higher omega-3 and omega-6 fatty acids.

Increased Energy Levels

My dog's energy levels also increased substantially. He began to show enthusiasm for activities he had previously been too lethargic to enjoy. His improved stamina indicated the nutritional value he was now receiving from his food. This was a dog reborn, living his life with a vitality I hadn't seen in years.

Better Digestive Health

Transitioning to a natural diet improved my dog's digestive health remarkably. He experienced less bloating and fewer episodes of gastric discomfort. His bowel movements became more regular and better formed, indicating a well-functioning digestive system.

Enhanced Immunity

My dog's immunity seemed to strengthen as well. He suffered fewer infections and reduced his recovery time from minor illnesses. The addition of fruits and vegetables in his diet meant he was consuming more antioxidants, which help fight off diseases.

Healthy Weight Management

Lastly, I noticed a positive change in my dog's weight. Being overweight had previously been a concern, with commercial foods often leading to overfeeding due to lower satiety. Natural food made it easier to manage his portion sizes, leading to a healthier weight.

Looking back, stretching to a natural diet was profound and undeniable. This chapter doesn't just recount these changes; it celebrates them. It's a testament to the power of a balanced, natural diet and how it can revitalize our pets' health.

To those considering making the switch, my advice is simple: leap. The improvements in your dog's health and happiness are worth it, and the journey is one you'll take together, strengthening the bond between you. You'll know you made the right choice with every wag of a healthy tail and every bound of renewed energy.

In the next chapter, we'll delve into the financial side of natural dog food, looking at cost versus benefit. Because ultimately, can you put a price on the health and happiness of your best friend?

8 The Financial Side: Cost Vs. Benefit Analysis Of Natural Dog Food

When considering a switch to natural dog food, one of the most significant concerns for many pet owners is the financial implication. The perception is that realistic or homemade dog food inevitably costs more than commercial kibble bought from the store. In this chapter, we delve into a cost-benefit analysis to dispel any misconceptions and give a clearer picture of what you can expect when choosing natural food for your pet.

Firstly, let's talk about the cost. The initial impression is that natural dog food is pricier - after all, quality ingredients often come with a higher price tag. However, this is only part of the story. The numbers can look different when you factor in the potential long-term savings.

The primary advantage of natural dog food lies in its contribution to your dog's health. Natural dog food often means less filler, fewer artificial additives, and more high-quality, nutritionally dense ingredients. This type of diet can help your dog maintain an ideal weight, reduce the risk of certain diseases, and improve overall vitality. The result? Fewer trips to the vet lowered medication costs and, potentially, a longer, happier life for your furry friend.

Think about it this way: investing in higher-quality food now could save on costly vet bills. This isn't to say that natural dog food will entirely prevent health issues, but it certainly contributes to a healthier lifestyle that can mitigate certain risks.

Then there's the question of preparation. If you make your dog's food at home, you might spend more time in the kitchen. This might be a drawback for some, but for others, it could be a cherished bonding time with their pet. And let's remember the potential savings from buying ingredients in bulk and using the same fresh produce you purchase for your meals.

Lastly, it's important to remember that every dog is different. What works for one might not work for another. The transition to natural dog food should be gradual and monitored closely to ensure your dog responds well.

In conclusion, while the upfront costs of natural dog food may be higher, the financial and health-related potential benefits make it a worthwhile investment. As pet owners, we want the best for our furry friends, including their diet. With a balanced view of the costs and benefits, you can make an informed decision about your dog's nutrition.

9 Frequently Asked Questions About Natural Dog Food

As more pet parents make the shift to natural food diets for their dogs, there are inevitably numerous questions that arise. In my journey, I've encountered a variety of inquiries - some from my research and others from fellow pet owners inspired by the changes they've seen in my dog. This chapter will address some of the most frequently asked questions about natural dog food.

Q1: What is considered "natural" dog food?

In the simplest terms, natural dog food typically refers to food free from artificial colors, flavors, preservatives, and by-products. It's often homemade, using fresh, high-quality ingredients that could include lean meats, fruits, vegetables, and whole grains.

Q2: Is natural dog food better for my dog than commercial dog food?

In many cases, yes. Like humans, dogs thrive on a balanced and varied diet. Natural foods often provide more essential nutrients, fiber, and moisture than commercial foods. It's important to note that every dog is different, and some may have specific dietary needs. Always consult a vet before making significant changes to your pet's diet.

Q3: Can I feed my dog the same natural foods I eat?

While many foods we eat can benefit dogs, it's crucial to remember that not all human foods are safe. Certain foods like chocolate, onions, grapes, and some sweeteners can be toxic to dogs. Always research or consult your vet if you need clarification on a particular food.

Q4: How do I transition my dog to a natural diet?

Transitioning should be done gradually to avoid upsetting your dog's digestive system. Start by replacing a small portion of their regular diet with natural food, gradually increasing the amount over a few weeks.

Q5: Is feeding a natural diet more expensive?

It can be, depending on the ingredients you choose. However, many dog owners find that the potential health benefits and reduced vet bills make it a worthy investment.

Remember, every dog is unique, and what works well for one might not work for another. Feeding your dog a natural diet is a personal decision that should be made considering your pet's specific health needs and lifestyle. It's always best to consult with a veterinarian before making any majoangesignificantyour dog's diet.

*Q6: Does this type of diet require supplementing his food?
Yes! Please talk your vet before any diet transition.

10 The Lasting Impact - Our Life Today On Natural Dog Food

As I write this chapter, Muttley, my ever-energetic pup, is playfully pawing at my feet, ready for our morning walk. There's an undeniable spark in his eyes and boundless energy in his gait - a vitality far less apparent before we embarked on our natural dog food journey. This newfound exuberance underscores the lasting impact of our decision to embrace a natural diet for Muttley.

From the moment we switched to natural dog food, the transformation in Muttley was notable. Once dull and lackluster, his coat began to shine and thicken into a luxurious, dense fur that rivals the finest of rugs. His energy levels, which had ebbed mid-day, are now consistent, fueling his desire for long walks and even longer play sessions.

His weight, an area of concern due to his breed's predisposition to obesity, stabilized within a healthy range. His stomach issues, an unpleasant yet frequent on a commercial diet, have all but vanished. The frequent regular, once a part of our routine, has significantly reduced. Today, his vet marveled at his health during his annual checkup, attributing it to his balanced, natural diet.

But the changes extend beyond the physical. There's an unmistakable joy in Muttley's demeanor and contentment that only comes from a diet that satisfies his hunger and his instinctive need for natural, wholesome food. He's more engaged during our training sessions, more responsive to our commands, and a happier, more well-adjusted companion overall.

Feeding Muttley natural dog food was not just a change in his diet but a commitment to enhancing his quality of life. Today, this decision reflects in his health, happiness, and the strong bond we've developed through our shared journey towards natural living.

The lasting impact of switching to natural dog food has extended beyond just Muttley and has influenced our approach to health and wellbeing. We've become more conscious of what goes into our bodies, more aware of the implications of processed food, and more dedicated to embracing a lifestyle that resonates with nature.

In closing this chapter, I look down at Muttley, who's now waiting patiently by the door, his tail wagging with anticipation. Our walk awaits, and with it, the promise of many more shared moments fueled by a lifestyle choice that's transformed not just his life but ours.

Switching to natural dog food was undoubtedly one of the best decisions we've made for Muttley. It's a choice that's brought healthier, happier days for our furry friend, with it, a lasting impact that's reshaped our lives for the better.

Conclusion - Lessons Learned From My Natural Dog Food Journey

As I sit here, pen in hand, I'm struck by how much I've learned on this journey toward a natural dog food diet. I'm more than just a dog owner now; I'm an informed advocate for my dog's well-being.

The initial decision to explore a natural diet for my dog was not without its challenges, but it was an enlightening and ultimately rewarding experience. What started as a simple choice has become a lifestyle change and a mission to ensure my furry friend enjoys the best health possible.

I've learned that every dog is unique. What works for one may not work for another, and there's no one-size-fits-all diet. Listening to your dog, observing his responses to different foods, and working with your veterinarian are vital steps in finding the best dietary plan for your pet.

My biggest revelation has been the direct connection between diet and overall health. The changes in my dog's energy levels, coat sheen, digestion, and general demeanor have been incredible. These improvements affirmed my belief that a natural diet could significantly impact a dog's quality of life.

While there were hurdles to overcome, I learned that preparation and persistence were vital. Transitioning from commercial food to a natural diet needed time and patience. Each small victory and each positive change was worth the effort, and the occasional setbacks were stepping stones leading us toward our goal.

Moreover, I realized that the financial investment in a natural diet reaped substantial returns in terms of health benefits. Fewer vet visits and less money spent on medication were proof enough that the 'cost' was a worthwhile investment.

The journey also taught me about community. I discovered a network of other pet owners striving to provide healthier lifestyles for their pets. Their advice, support, and shared experiences were invaluable.

Finally, the most poignant lesson has been about love. This journey wasn't just about changing a diet. It was about profoundly expressing my love for my dog: investing time, effort, and resources to enhance his health and happiness.

To those considering a similar journey, remember that it's a process of exploration and learning. Start small, arm yourself with knowledge, and keep your dog's best interests at heart. The journey may be challenging, but the rewards are priceless.

Reflecting on our journey, I am grateful for the lessons learned and improvements. The path to natural dog food has been much more than a dietary change; it has been a journey of love, commitment, and an ongoing quest for wellness. This is the legacy I want to leave for other dog owners, an affirmation that the natural path is not only possible but also incredibly rewarding.

Appendix: Recommended Resources For Further Reading

As a devoted dog owner, I understand the importance of continuous learning. The journey to natural dog food I've shared in this book evolved, much of it spurred by further readings and constant research. The world of canine nutrition is vast and complex, and understanding it thoroughly requires an ongoing commitment to learning.

In this section, I'd like to share some books, websites, online forums, and other resources that have helped me. While my journey was specific to my dog's needs and our shared experiences, these resources provide broader perspectives and deeper insights into the world of natural dog nutrition that can benefit any dog owner considering this path.

Books:

1. "The Nature of Animal Healing" by Martin Goldstein, D.V.M.
2. "Dr. Pitcairn's Complete Guide to Natural Health for Dogs & Cats" by Richard H. Pitcairn and Susan Hubble Pitcairn
3. "Raw and Natural Nutrition for Dogs" by Lew Olson, Ph.D.
4. "The Barf Diet" by Ian Billinghurst

Websites:

1. Whole Dog Journal (www.wholedogjournal.com): This site offers a wealth of articles on all aspects of dog care, including nutrition, and has an excellent section on natural and homemade diets.
2. Dog Food Advisor (www.dogfoodadvisor.com): An excellent resource for understanding commercial.
3. dog food and exploring healthier alternatives.
4. The Possible Canine (www.thepossiblecanine.com): Run by a canine nutritionist, this blog covers a wide range of dog nutrition and health topics.

Online Forums:

1. Raw Feeding Community (www.rawfeedingcommunity.com): This forum is a great place to connect with other dog owners who feed their dogs a natural diet.
2. Dogster Raw Feeding Diet Forum (www.dogster.com):
3. Another excellent forum to connect with experienced raw feeders and natural dog food enthusiasts.

**Documentaries: **

1. "Pet Fooled" - Available on various streaming platforms, this documentary provides an in-depth look at the pet food industry.
2. "The Dog Cancer Series: Rethinking the Canine Epidemic" -A film that explores the potential link between commercial pet food and dog cancer.

Remember, each dog is unique, and what works for one may not work for another. It's essential to consult with your vet or a canine nutrition expert when making significant changes to your dog's diet. These resources are not a substitute for professional advice but are tools that can help inform your conversations with professionals and enhance your understanding of your dog's nutritional needs.

Your journey with your dog is your own. Use these resources as a starting point, but always listen to your dog and seek professional advice when needed. The journey towards better canine health and wellness through natural food is rewarding, and I wish you and your furry friend the best of luck.